Summary

> **Introduction to the Vegetarian Diet and Reasons for Adopting It**: This book begins by exploring the many compelling reasons to adopt a vegetarian diet. It delves into the health benefits, ethical considerations, and positive environmental impacts, providing readers with a comprehensive understanding of why this lifestyle choice is both beneficial and meaningful.

> **Practical Guide to Transitioning to a Vegetarian Diet**: Transitioning to a vegetarian diet can seem daunting, but this guide offers practical, step-by-step advice to make the change smooth and enjoyable. Topics include how to gradually reduce meat consumption, find satisfying plant-based alternatives, and adapt favorite recipes to be vegetarian-friendly.

- **Planning Balanced and Nutritious Meals**: Ensuring a vegetarian diet is balanced and nutritious requires careful planning. This section provides detailed guidelines on composing meals that meet all nutritional needs, emphasizing the importance of including a variety of foods to achieve a well-rounded diet.

- **Creative and Nutritious Vegetarian Recipes for Every Meal**: Discover a diverse collection of delicious vegetarian recipes designed for every meal of the day. From energizing breakfasts to hearty dinners, these recipes showcase the versatility and richness of vegetarian cuisine, proving that plant-based eating can be both satisfying and exciting.

- **Information on Protein-Rich Foods**: Contrary to common misconceptions, there are numerous plant-based sources of protein. This chapter highlights the best protein-rich foods, explaining how to incorporate them into your diet to meet your daily protein requirements effectively.

➢ **Tips for Maintaining Nutritional Balance and Facing the Day with Energy**: Maintaining high energy levels and overall well-being is crucial. This section offers practical tips on how to structure meals and snacks throughout the day to ensure a steady intake of essential nutrients, helping you stay energized and focused.

➢ **Insights into Sources of Nutrients Such as Iron, Calcium, Vitamins**: A well-planned vegetarian diet can provide all necessary nutrients. This chapter provides in-depth information on the best plant-based sources of essential nutrients like iron, calcium, and vitamins B12 and D, along with tips on how to optimize their absorption.

➢ **Tips for Shopping and Reading Nutritional Labels**: Navigating the grocery store can be a breeze with the right knowledge. This section offers practical advice on choosing nutrient-dense foods, understanding nutritional labels, and making informed decisions to support a healthy vegetarian diet.

➢ **Tips for Overcoming Social Challenges**: Eating vegetarian in a predominantly meat-eating world can present social challenges. This chapter provides strategies for communicating your dietary choices, dealing with social pressure, and finding support within a community of like-minded individuals.

➢ **Impact of the Vegetarian Diet on Health, the Environment, and the Body**: The book concludes by reflecting on the long-term benefits of a vegetarian diet. It examines the positive effects on personal health, the significant reduction in environmental footprint, and the overall improvement in physical well-being, illustrating how mindful eating can contribute to a healthier, more sustainable world.

<u>Benefits for book buyers:</u>

- Increased awareness of health benefits;

- Ability to successfully adopt and maintain a healthy lifestyle;

- Improved overall health;

- Access to delicious recipes and practical tips;

- Support in the transition to a style.

<u>Things people will learn to do by reading the book:</u>

- Choose and prepare balanced and healthy vegetarian meals;

- Get the protein and nutrients you need without meat or fish,

- Plan weekly meals with various recipes;

- Develop conscious eating habits,

- Contribute to greater environmental sustainability.

Introduction to the Vegetarian Diet: Exploring Motivations for a Meat-Free Lifestyle

In an age where health consciousness and ethical considerations are becoming increasingly paramount, the vegetarian diet has emerged not only as a culinary trend but as a profound lifestyle choice. This dietary regimen, which eschews the consumption of meat, fish, and poultry, is embraced by millions worldwide. However, the motivations behind this shift extend far beyond the confines of the kitchen, encompassing a rich tapestry of personal, ethical, environmental, and health-related reasons.

At its core, the vegetarian diet is rooted in a philosophy that values the sanctity of all living beings. For many, this diet represents a compassionate stance against the industrial practices that dominate modern meat production, practices often criticized for their cruelty towards animals. By choosing to abstain from meat, vegetarians aim to reduce animal suffering and promote a more humane world.

Beyond ethical considerations, environmental concerns drive a significant portion of the population towards vegetarianism. The meat industry is a known contributor to a range of environmental issues, from deforestation and water pollution to greenhouse gas emissions. As awareness of climate change and ecological degradation grows, so too does the appeal of a plant-based diet that promises a lower carbon footprint and a more sustainable future.

Health benefits also play a crucial role in the decision to adopt a vegetarian diet. Numerous studies have highlighted the potential health advantages of a diet rich in fruits, vegetables, legumes, and whole grains. From reducing the risk of chronic diseases such as heart disease, diabetes, and certain cancers to promoting overall longevity and well-being, the scientific community increasingly recognizes the virtues of vegetarianism.

Furthermore, cultural and spiritual beliefs often intertwine with dietary choices. In various traditions and religions around the world, vegetarianism is seen as a path to spiritual purity and enlightenment, reflecting a deep-seated connection between diet and inner well-being.

In essence, the vegetarian diet is far more than a mere avoidance of meat; it is a deliberate, multifaceted choice that resonates with a broad spectrum of values and beliefs.

Whether driven by a desire for better health, a commitment to environmental stewardship, ethical convictions, or spiritual fulfillment, the journey towards vegetarianism is a testament to the profound ways in which our food choices shape our lives and the world around us.

Transitioning to a vegetarian diet can be a transformative and enriching experience, offering numerous benefits for your health, the environment, and animal welfare. However, making the switch from a meat-based diet to a plant-based one can seem daunting at first. This practical guide aims to provide you with a step-by-step approach to ease your transition and help you embrace a vegetarian lifestyle with confidence and joy.

1. Educate Yourself

Before embarking on your vegetarian journey, take the time to educate yourself about the basics of vegetarian nutrition. Understand the different types of vegetarian diets, such as lacto-vegetarian, ovo-vegetarian, and vegan, and decide which one suits your lifestyle and preferences. Familiarize yourself with essential nutrients that need special attention in a vegetarian diet, such as protein, iron, calcium, vitamin B12, and omega-3 fatty acids.

2. Start Slow

Making a sudden, drastic change to your diet can be overwhelming. Instead, start slow by incorporating more plant-based meals into your weekly routine. Begin with Meatless Mondays, gradually increasing the number of meat-free days as you become more comfortable with vegetarian cooking. This gradual approach allows your palate and digestive system to adjust smoothly.

3. Plan Balanced Meals

Ensure that your meals are balanced and nutritious by including a variety of food groups. A typical vegetarian plate should include:

- **Protein**: Beans, lentils, tofu, tempeh, chickpeas, and quinoa.

- **Healthy Fats**: Avocados, nuts, seeds, and olive oil.

- **Complex Carbohydrates**: Whole grains like brown rice, oats, barley, and whole-wheat products.

- **Fruits and Vegetables**: A colorful array of seasonal and diverse produce.

- **Dairy or Dairy Alternatives**: Milk, cheese, yogurt, or fortified plant-based alternatives.

4. Discover New Recipes

One of the joys of transitioning to a vegetarian diet is exploring new recipes and cuisines. Experiment with dishes from different cultures that naturally emphasize plant-based ingredients. Try Mediterranean falafel, Indian lentil curry, Mexican black bean tacos, or Italian eggplant Parmesan. There are countless vegetarian cookbooks and online resources to inspire your culinary adventures.

5. Stock Your Pantry

A well-stocked pantry makes it easier to prepare vegetarian meals. Keep essentials like canned beans, lentils, whole grains, nuts, seeds, spices, and herbs on hand. Fresh fruits and vegetables, tofu, tempeh, and dairy or plant-based alternatives should be regular staples in your refrigerator.

6. Focus on Nutrient-Dense Foods

While transitioning, ensure that you're consuming nutrient-dense foods to meet your dietary needs. Include sources of iron (spinach, lentils), calcium (broccoli, fortified plant milks), vitamin B12 (fortified cereals, supplements), and omega-3 fatty acids (chia seeds, walnuts).

7. Connect with a Community

Joining a community of like-minded individuals can provide support and motivation. Engage with online forums, local vegetarian groups, or social media communities where you can share experiences, ask questions, and find inspiration. Many people find it easier to stick to dietary changes when they have a supportive network.

8. Listen to Your Body

Pay attention to how your body responds to the new diet. While many people experience positive changes such as increased energy and improved digestion, it's important to listen to your body and make adjustments as needed. If you

16

have any concerns, consider consulting with a registered dietitian who specializes in vegetarian nutrition.

9. Be Mindful of Dining Out

Dining out as a vegetarian can be challenging, but it's becoming easier with the growing popularity of plant-based diets. Research restaurant menus in advance, and don't hesitate to ask for vegetarian options or modifications. Many establishments are happy to accommodate dietary preferences.

10. Celebrate Your Progress

Transitioning to a vegetarian diet is a significant achievement. Celebrate your progress and milestones along the way. Acknowledge the positive impact your choices have on your health, the environment, and animal welfare.

Remember, it's okay to make mistakes and learn from them as you continue your journey.

By following this practical guide, you'll find that transitioning to a vegetarian diet can be a rewarding and enjoyable process. Embrace the adventure, savor the new flavors, and take pride in the positive changes you're making for yourself and the world around you.

Balanced and Nutritious Vegetarian Meal Planning

Planning balanced and nutritious meals is essential to ensure that your vegetarian diet meets all your nutritional needs. This guide will help you create a well-rounded meal plan that incorporates a variety of food groups, ensuring you get the essential nutrients for optimal health. Let's break it down into breakfast, lunch, dinner, and snacks.

Breakfast

1. Smoothie Bowl

- Ingredients:

  - 1 banana

  - 1 cup spinach

  - 1/2 cup frozen berries

  - 1/2 cup almond milk

- 1 tablespoon chia seeds

- 1 tablespoon almond butter

- Toppings: sliced fruits, granola, nuts

- Nutritional Highlights:

  - Rich in vitamins A, C, and K from spinach and berries

  - Protein and healthy fats from almond butter and chia
seeds

- Fiber from fruits and chia seeds

2. Avocado Toast with a Twist

- Ingredients:

  - 1 slice whole-grain bread

  - 1/2 avocado

  - 1 poached egg (optional for ovo-vegetarians)

  - Cherry tomatoes, halved

- A sprinkle of hemp seeds

- Salt, pepper, and a dash of lemon juice

- Nutritional Highlights:

- Healthy fats from avocado

- Protein from the egg and hemp seeds

- Fiber from whole-grain bread

- Vitamins and antioxidants from tomatoes

Lunch

1. Quinoa and Black Bean Salad

-Ingredients:

- 1 cup cooked quinoa

- 1/2 cup black beans, rinsed and drained

- 1/2 cup corn kernels

- 1 red bell pepper, diced

- 1/4 cup red onion, finely chopped

- 1/4 cup cilantro, chopped

- Dressing: olive oil, lime juice, cumin, salt, and pepper

- Nutritional Highlights:

  - Complete protein from quinoa and black beans

  - Fiber and vitamins from vegetables

  - Healthy fats from olive oil

2. Lentil and Vegetable Stir-Fry

- Ingredients:

  - 1 cup cooked lentils

  - 1 cup broccoli florets

  - 1 carrot, sliced

  - 1 bell pepper, sliced

  - 1/2 cup snap peas

- 2 tablespoons soy sauce

- 1 tablespoon sesame oil

- 1 teaspoon grated ginger

- 1 garlic clove, minced

- Brown rice or whole-grain noodles to serve

- Nutritional Highlights:

- Protein and iron from lentils

- A wide range of vitamins and minerals from assorted vegetables

- Fiber from brown rice or whole-grain noodles

Dinner

1. Chickpea and Spinach Curry

- Ingredients:

- 1 can chickpeas, rinsed and drained

- 1 cup spinach, chopped

- 1 onion, diced

- 2 garlic cloves, minced

- 1 can coconut milk

- 2 tablespoons curry powder

- 1 teaspoon turmeric

- Salt and pepper to taste

- Brown rice or quinoa to serve

-Nutritional Highlights:

  - Protein and fiber from chickpeas

  - Iron and calcium from spinach

- Healthy fats from coconut milk

2. Stuffed Bell Peppers

- Ingredients:

- 4 bell peppers, tops cut off and seeds removed

- 1 cup cooked brown rice

- 1 cup black beans, rinsed and drained

- 1 cup corn kernels

- 1 cup diced tomatoes

- 1/2 cup shredded cheese (optional for lacto-vegetarians)

- Spices: cumin, paprika, salt, and pepper

-Nutritional Highlights:

- Complete protein from rice and beans

- Vitamins A and C from bell peppers

- Fiber from beans and corn

Snacks

1. Hummus and Veggie Sticks

- Ingredients:

  - 1/2 cup hummus

  - Carrot sticks

  - Celery sticks

  - Cucumber slices

  - Bell pepper slices

- Nutritional Highlights:

  - Protein and healthy fats from hummus

  - Vitamins and fiber from vegetables

2. Greek Yogurt with Nuts and Berries

- Ingredients:

  - 1 cup Greek yogurt

  - 1/4 cup mixed nuts (almonds, walnuts, cashews)

    - 1/2 cup mixed berries (blueberries, strawberries, raspberries)

- Nutritional Highlights:

  - Protein and probiotics from Greek yogurt

  - Healthy fats from nuts

- Antioxidants and vitamins from berries

Tips for Balanced Meal Planning

1.Variety is Key: Ensure a variety of foods to cover all nutrient bases.

2. Focus on Whole Foods: Prioritize whole, minimally processed foods for maximum nutrition.

3. Stay Hydrated: Drink plenty of water throughout the day.

4.Mind Your Portions: Pay attention to portion sizes to avoid overeating or undereating.

5.Listen to Your Body: Adjust your meal plan based on how your body feels and responds.

By incorporating these balanced and nutritious meals into your daily routine, you can enjoy a vibrant, healthful vegetarian diet that supports your overall well-being.

Creative and Nutritious Vegetarian Recipes for Every Meal

Embracing a vegetarian lifestyle opens up a world of culinary creativity and nutritional abundance. Here are delicious and balanced vegetarian recipes to inspire you from breakfast to dinner, ensuring you enjoy every meal while nourishing your body with wholesome ingredients.

Breakfast: Savory Chickpea Flour Pancakes with Avocado Salsa

Ingredients:

- For Chickpea Flour Pancakes:

  - 1 cup chickpea flour

  - 1 cup water

  - 1/2 teaspoon baking powder

  - Salt and pepper to taste

  - 1 tablespoon olive oil

- For Avocado Salsa:

  - 1 ripe avocado, diced

  - 1 small tomato, diced

  - 1/4 cup red onion, finely chopped

  - 1/4 cup fresh cilantro, chopped

  - Juice of 1 lime

  - Salt and pepper to taste

Instructions:

1. In a bowl, whisk together chickpea flour, water, baking powder, salt, and pepper until smooth.

2. Heat olive oil in a non-stick skillet over medium heat. Pour about 1/4 cup of batter into the skillet and spread it into a circle.

3. Cook until bubbles form on the surface and the edges start to lift, then flip and cook the other side until golden brown. Repeat with remaining batter.

4. Meanwhile, prepare the avocado salsa by mixing diced avocado, tomato, red onion, cilantro, lime juice, salt, and pepper in a bowl.

5. Serve chickpea flour pancakes topped with avocado salsa. Enjoy your savory and satisfying breakfast!

Lunch: Mediterranean Stuffed Sweet Potatoes

Ingredients:

- 2 large sweet potatoes

- 1 cup cooked quinoa

- 1 can chickpeas, rinsed and drained

- 1/2 cucumber, diced

- 1/2 cup cherry tomatoes, halved

- 1/4 cup Kalamata olives, sliced

- 1/4 cup red onion, finely chopped

- 1/4 cup crumbled feta cheese (optional for lacto-vegetarians)

- Juice of 1 lemon

- 2 tablespoons olive oil

- 1 teaspoon dried oregano

- Salt and pepper to taste

Instructions:

1. Preheat oven to 400°F (200°C). Wash sweet potatoes and prick them several times with a fork. Place them on a baking sheet and bake for 45-60 minutes, or until tender.

2. In a large bowl, combine cooked quinoa, chickpeas, cucumber, cherry tomatoes, Kalamata olives, red onion, and feta cheese (if using).

3. In a small bowl, whisk together lemon juice, olive oil,

dried oregano, salt, and pepper. Pour over the quinoa mixture and toss to coat.

4. Cut open each sweet potato lengthwise and fluff the flesh with a fork. Spoon the quinoa mixture into the sweet potatoes.

5. Garnish with additional crumbled feta cheese and fresh herbs if desired. Serve warm and enjoy these Mediterranean-inspired stuffed sweet potatoes!

Dinner: Thai Red Curry with Tofu and Vegetables

Ingredients:

- 1 block firm tofu, pressed and cubed

- 1 tablespoon vegetable oil

- 1 onion, thinly sliced

- 2 bell peppers (any color), sliced

- 1 zucchini, sliced

- 1 cup broccoli florets

- 1 can (14 oz) coconut milk

- 2-3 tablespoons Thai red curry paste (adjust to taste)

- 1 tablespoon soy sauce or tamari

- 1 tablespoon brown sugar or coconut sugar

- Juice of 1 lime

- Fresh basil or cilantro for garnish

- Cooked rice or noodles for serving

Instructions:

1. Heat vegetable oil in a large skillet or wok over medium-high heat. Add cubed tofu and cook until golden brown on all sides. Remove tofu from skillet and set aside.

2. In the same skillet, add sliced onion and cook until softened. Add bell peppers, zucchini, and broccoli florets, and stir-fry for 3-4 minutes until vegetables are crisp-tender.

3. Stir in Thai red curry paste and cook for 1 minute until fragrant.

4. Pour in coconut milk, soy sauce or tamari, and brown sugar. Bring to a simmer and cook for 5-7 minutes until vegetables are cooked through and the sauce has thickened slightly.

5. Add cooked tofu back to the skillet and stir gently to combine. Cook for another 2-3 minutes to heat through.

6. Remove from heat and stir in lime juice. Taste and adjust seasoning if needed.

7. Serve Thai red curry over cooked rice or noodles. Garnish with fresh basil or cilantro. Enjoy this aromatic and flavorful dinner!

Snack: Mango Coconut Chia Pudding

Ingredients:

- 1/4 cup chia seeds

- 1 cup coconut milk (or any plant-based milk)

- 1 ripe mango, diced

- 1 tablespoon shredded coconut (optional)

- Honey or maple syrup to taste (optional)

Instructions:

1. In a bowl or jar, mix chia seeds and coconut milk. Stir well to combine. Let it sit for 10 minutes, then stir again to prevent clumping.

2. Cover and refrigerate for at least 2 hours or overnight until the chia seeds have absorbed the liquid and the mixture has thickened to a pudding-like consistency.

3. Before serving, layer the chia pudding with diced mango in serving glasses or bowls.

4. Optionally, sprinkle shredded coconut on top and drizzle with honey or maple syrup for added sweetness.

5. Enjoy this refreshing and nutrient-packed mango coconut chia pudding as a satisfying snack!

These creative and nutritious vegetarian recipes showcase the diverse flavors and health benefits of plant-based eating. Whether you're enjoying a hearty breakfast, a vibrant lunch, a flavorful dinner, or a wholesome snack, these recipes will delight your taste buds and nourish your body. Happy cooking and eating!

Protein-Rich Vegetarian Foods: A Comprehensive Guide

Maintaining a vegetarian diet while ensuring adequate protein intake is crucial for overall health, muscle maintenance, and metabolic functions. Fortunately, a variety of plant-based foods are rich in protein and can easily meet dietary needs. Here's a guide to some of the best vegetarian protein sources:

1. Legumes

Beans: Black beans, kidney beans, chickpeas, and lentils are excellent sources of protein. A cup of cooked lentils, for instance, provides around 18 grams of protein.

Peas: Green peas offer about 8 grams of protein per cup. Split peas, used in soups, are also protein-rich.

2. Soy Products

Tofu: Made from soybean curds, tofu is a versatile ingredient that can be used in a variety of dishes. A 100-gram serving contains about 8 grams of protein.

Tempeh: Fermented soybeans form tempeh, which has a nutty flavor and firm texture. It offers about 19 grams of protein per 100 grams.

Edamame: Young soybeans, either fresh or frozen, are often served as a snack or in salads and contain 17 grams of protein per cup.

3. Nuts and Seeds

Almonds: A 28-gram serving (about 23 almonds) provides 6 grams of protein.

Chia Seeds: These tiny seeds pack 4 grams of protein per 28 grams (2 tablespoons), along with a good dose of fiber and omega-3 fatty acids.

Pumpkin Seeds: Also known as pepitas, they offer around 7 grams of protein per 28 grams.

Hemp Seeds: Containing all nine essential amino acids, hemp seeds provide 10 grams of protein per 28 grams.

4. Grains

Quinoa: Unlike most grains, quinoa is a complete protein, meaning it contains all nine essential amino acids. One cup of cooked quinoa has about 8 grams of protein.

Farro: This ancient grain provides about 6 grams of protein per cup cooked.

Oats: A versatile breakfast staple, oats offer 6 grams of protein per cup when cooked.

5. Dairy and Dairy Alternatives

Greek Yogurt: A cup of Greek yogurt can provide between 10 to 20 grams of protein, depending on the brand and fat content.

Cottage Cheese: This fresh cheese curd product offers around 14 grams of protein per half-cup serving.

Milk and Milk Alternatives: Cow's milk provides 8 grams of protein per cup. Fortified plant-based milks, such as soy or pea milk, can offer similar protein content.

6. Vegetables

Spinach: While not as high in protein as legumes or soy, spinach offers a respectable 5 grams of protein per cooked cup.

Broccoli: This cruciferous vegetable provides 4 grams of protein per cup when cooked.

7. Meat Substitutes

Seitan: Made from wheat gluten, seitan is a popular meat substitute that offers an impressive 25 grams of protein per 100 grams.

Veggie Burgers and Sausages: Many commercial products are fortified with protein and can provide about 10-15 grams per serving. Always check the labels for specific protein content.

Combining Foods for Complete Proteins

While many plant-based foods provide significant protein, not all are complete proteins. Combining different sources, such as beans with rice or hummus with whole grain bread, can ensure you get all essential amino acids.

Tips for Increasing Protein Intake

- **Snacking:** Incorporate protein-rich snacks like nuts, seeds, and Greek yogurt.

- **Cooking:** Add beans to soups, salads, and casseroles.

- **Breakfast:** Start the day with protein-packed meals like oatmeal topped with nuts and seeds or a smoothie with Greek yogurt and protein powder.

- **Supplements:** Consider protein powders made from peas, hemp, or soy for an extra boost.

With a wide array of protein-rich vegetarian options available, it's easy to meet daily protein needs while enjoying a varied and delicious diet. Balancing different sources and incorporating them into meals throughout the

day can ensure you get the essential nutrients for a healthy

lifestyle.

***Tips for maintaining nutritional balance and facing the day with energy.**￼*

Maintaining nutritional balance as a vegetarian and ensuring you face the day with energy requires careful planning and knowledge about key nutrients. Here are some tips to help you thrive on a vegetarian diet:

1. Embrace Variety

- **Diversify Your Plate:** Incorporate a wide range of fruits, vegetables, whole grains, legumes, nuts, and seeds to ensure a broad spectrum of nutrients.

- **Colorful Diet:** Eating a rainbow of colorful foods can help you get a variety of vitamins and minerals.

2. Focus on Protein

- **Plant-Based Proteins:** Include sources such as beans, lentils, chickpeas, tofu, tempeh, edamame, quinoa, and seitan.

- **Complementary Proteins:** Combine foods like rice and beans or hummus and whole wheat pita to get a complete amino acid profile.

3. Prioritize Iron Intake

- **Iron-Rich Foods:** Eat spinach, lentils, chickpeas, quinoa, fortified cereals, and pumpkin seeds.

- **Enhance Absorption:** Pair iron-rich foods with vitamin C sources like citrus fruits, bell peppers, and tomatoes to boost absorption.

4. Ensure Adequate Vitamin B12

- **Fortified Foods:** Consume fortified plant milks, cereals, and nutritional yeast to get enough B12.

- **Supplements:** Consider taking a B12 supplement, as this vitamin is primarily found in animal products.

5. Get Enough Calcium

- **Calcium Sources:** Eat leafy greens like kale and bok choy, fortified plant milks, almonds, and sesame seeds.

- **Bioavailability:** Note that some greens like spinach contain oxalates, which can inhibit calcium absorption. Rotate different sources for better bioavailability.

6. Omega-3 Fatty Acids

- **Plant Sources:** Include flaxseeds, chia seeds, walnuts, and hemp seeds in your diet.

- **ALA to DHA Conversion:** Your body converts ALA (plant-based omega-3) to DHA and EPA. Consider algae-based supplements for a direct source of DHA.

47

7. Zinc and Magnesium

- **Zinc:** Include beans, lentils, chickpeas, nuts, seeds, and whole grains.

- **Magnesium:** Incorporate foods like dark leafy greens, bananas, avocados, nuts, seeds, and whole grains.

8. Stay Hydrated

- **Water Intake:** Drink plenty of water throughout the day to stay hydrated.

- **Hydrating Foods:** Eat water-rich fruits and vegetables like cucumbers, watermelon, oranges, and strawberries.

9. Plan Your Meals

- **Balanced Meals:** Ensure each meal includes a mix of macronutrients (carbohydrates, proteins, fats) and micronutrients.

- **Snacks:** Keep healthy snacks like nuts, seeds, fruit, and veggie sticks handy for sustained energy levels.

10. Listen to Your Body

- **Energy Levels:** Pay attention to how different foods make you feel and adjust your diet accordingly.

- **Consult Professionals:** Periodically consult with a dietitian or nutritionist to tailor your diet to your individual needs.

Sample Daily Meal Plan

Breakfast

- **Smoothie:** Blend spinach, banana, chia seeds, almond milk, and a scoop of protein powder.

- **Whole Grain Toast:** Top with avocado and a sprinkle of nutritional yeast.

Lunch

- **Quinoa Salad:** Mix quinoa with black beans, corn, tomatoes, avocado, and a lime vinaigrette.

- **Side of Fruit:** A bowl of mixed berries.

Snack

- **Trail Mix:** A handful of nuts, seeds, and dried fruit.

- **Carrot Sticks:** With hummus for dipping.

Dinner

- **Stir-Fry:** Tofu with broccoli, bell peppers, carrots, and snap peas over brown rice.

- **Leafy Green Salad:** Mixed greens with a tahini dressing.

Evening Snack

- **Yogurt:** A serving of fortified plant-based yogurt with a sprinkle of granola.

By following these tips and paying attention to your body's needs, you can maintain a well-balanced vegetarian diet that keeps you energized and healthy.

Nourishing Nutrients: A Vegetarian's Guide to Iron, Calcium, and Vitamins

Embracing a vegetarian lifestyle can be both a rewarding and healthful choice, but it requires mindful planning to ensure adequate intake of essential nutrients. Among these, iron, calcium, and various vitamins play pivotal roles in maintaining overall health. Here's a comprehensive guide to vegetarian-friendly sources of these crucial nutrients.

Iron

Iron is essential for producing hemoglobin, a protein in red blood cells that carries oxygen throughout the body. While meat is a well-known source of iron, vegetarians can obtain this nutrient from various plant-based foods.

1. **Legumes and Pulses**: Lentils, chickpeas, and beans are excellent sources of non-heme iron. Incorporating

dishes like lentil soup, chickpea salads, and bean stews can boost iron intake.

2. **Dark Leafy Greens**: Spinach, kale, and Swiss chard are not only rich in iron but also packed with other vitamins and minerals. Adding these greens to smoothies, salads, or stir-fries can enhance nutrient intake.

3. **Fortified Foods**: Many cereals, bread, and plant-based milks are fortified with iron. Checking labels can help identify these iron-rich options.

4. **Nuts and Seeds**: Pumpkin seeds, sesame seeds, and cashews are good sources of iron. Snacking on these or adding them to meals can be beneficial.

5. **Whole Grains**: Quinoa, brown rice, and oatmeal are not only nutritious but also contain iron. They can be used as a base for various dishes.

Calcium

Calcium is vital for strong bones and teeth, muscle function, and nerve signaling. While dairy products are well-known calcium sources, there are plenty of plant-based options available for vegetarians.

1. **Fortified Plant Milks**: Almond milk, soy milk, and oat milk often have added calcium. These can be used in smoothies, cereals, and baking.

2. **Tofu and Tempeh**: These soy-based products are not only high in protein but also fortified with calcium. They can be incorporated into stir-fries, salads, and sandwiches.

3. **Leafy Greens**: Collard greens, bok choy, and broccoli are excellent sources of calcium. They can be steamed, sautéed, or added to soups.

4. **Almonds**: These nuts are not only nutritious but also a good source of calcium. Enjoy them as a snack or add them to salads and desserts.

5. **Fortified Juices and Cereals**: Orange juice and cereals fortified with calcium can help meet daily requirements. Always check the labels to ensure they provide adequate calcium.

Vitamins

Vitamins are essential for numerous bodily functions, from maintaining healthy skin to supporting the immune system. Here are key vitamins and their vegetarian sources:

1. **Vitamin B12**: This vitamin is crucial for nerve function and blood formation but is not naturally found in plant foods. Vegetarians can obtain B12 from

fortified cereals, plant milks, and nutritional yeast. Supplements are also a reliable source.

2. **Vitamin D**: Essential for calcium absorption and bone health, Vitamin D can be obtained from fortified foods such as plant milks and orange juice. Sun exposure also helps the body produce Vitamin D, but supplements might be necessary, especially in less sunny regions.

3. **Vitamin C**: This vitamin boosts the immune system and aids in iron absorption. Citrus fruits, strawberries, bell peppers, and broccoli are rich in Vitamin C and can be easily incorporated into a vegetarian diet.

4. **Vitamin A**: Important for vision and immune function, Vitamin A can be found in carrots, sweet potatoes, spinach, and kale. These vegetables can be included in various dishes to ensure adequate intake.

5. **Vitamin E**: An antioxidant that helps protect cells from damage, Vitamin E can be found in nuts, seeds, spinach, and broccoli. Including these foods in meals and snacks can help meet Vitamin E needs.

A well-planned vegetarian diet can provide all the necessary nutrients, including iron, calcium, and vitamins, essential for optimal health. By incorporating a diverse range of plant-based foods and fortified products, vegetarians can enjoy a balanced and nutritious diet that supports their overall well-being.

Tips for shopping and reading nutritional labels

Shopping as a vegetarian involves careful planning and reading nutrition labels to ensure a balanced diet. Here are some tips to help you navigate the grocery store and make informed choices:

1. **Plan Your Meals**:

   - Create a weekly meal plan to ensure you have a variety of nutrients.

   - Make a shopping list based on your meal plan to avoid impulse buying and ensure you have all necessary ingredients.

2. **Shop the Perimeter**:

   - Focus on the outer edges of the grocery store where fresh produce, dairy, and whole foods are usually located.

- Avoid processed foods found in the center aisles whenever possible.

3. **Include a Variety of Protein Sources**:

   - Incorporate legumes (beans, lentils, chickpeas), tofu, tempeh, seitan, and edamame.

   - Include dairy or dairy alternatives like milk, yogurt, and cheese if you consume them.

4. **Stock Up on Whole Grains**:

   - Opt for whole grains like brown rice, quinoa, oats, barley, and whole wheat products.

5. **Choose a Rainbow of Fruits and Vegetables**:

- Aim for a variety of colors to ensure a wide range of vitamins and minerals.

6. **Healthy Fats**:

- Include sources of healthy fats such as avocados, nuts, seeds, and olive oil.

7. **Watch for Fortified Foods**:

- Look for foods fortified with vitamins and minerals like B12, iron, calcium, and vitamin D, which are sometimes lacking in vegetarian diets.

Reading Nutrition Labels

1. **Check Serving Size**:

   - Ensure the serving size on the label matches the amount you actually consume. All the nutritional information is based on this serving size.

2. **Look at the Ingredients List**:

   - Ingredients are listed by weight, from highest to lowest. The first few ingredients are the most prominent in the product.

   - Avoid products with long lists of ingredients, especially those with unrecognizable or highly processed items.

3. **Protein Content**:

   - Aim for products with a good source of
     protein, especially if they are part of your main
     meals or snacks.

4. **Watch for Hidden Animal Products**:

   - Be aware of non-vegetarian ingredients like
     gelatin, rennet, or certain additives derived
     from animals.

5. **Check for Added Sugars**:

   - Limit products with high amounts of added
     sugars. Look for terms like sucrose, high
     fructose corn syrup, and cane sugar.

6. **Evaluate Fiber Content**:

   - Choose products high in dietary fiber, which is important for digestion and overall health.

7. **Watch Sodium Levels**:

   - Monitor the sodium content, especially in canned and processed foods, to avoid excessive salt intake.

8. **Vitamins and Minerals**:

   - Check for essential nutrients like iron, calcium, vitamin D, and B12. Fortified foods can help fill nutritional gaps.

9. **Understand Nutrient Claims**:

- Terms like "low-fat," "light," "organic," or "natural" have specific meanings regulated by health authorities. Know what these terms mean to make informed choices.

Additional Tips

- **Buy Seasonal and Local**: Seasonal produce is often fresher and more affordable. Farmers' markets are a great place to find local and seasonal options.

- **Consider Frozen and Canned Options**: These can be just as nutritious as fresh and have a longer shelf life. Look for options without added sugars or salt.

- **Experiment with New Foods**: Try different types of grains, legumes, and vegetables to keep your diet interesting and nutrient-rich.

- **Read Up on Vegetarian Nutrition**: Educate yourself about the nutrients you need to pay attention to and how to incorporate them into your diet.

By following these tips, you can ensure a nutritious, balanced vegetarian diet while making the most of your grocery shopping experience.

A vegetarian diet can have profound impacts on health, the environment, and the body. Here's a detailed look at each aspect.

1. **Nutritional Benefits**:

   • **Rich in Nutrients**: A well-planned vegetarian diet can provide all the essential nutrients, including vitamins, minerals, and fiber, often through a higher intake of fruits, vegetables, legumes, nuts, and whole grains.

   • **Heart Health**: Vegetarian diets are typically lower in saturated fats and cholesterol, which can lead to lower blood pressure, reduced risk of heart disease, and improved cholesterol levels.

   • **Weight Management**: Vegetarians often have a lower body mass index (BMI) and are less likely to be overweight or obese, due to higher intake of fiber-rich foods and lower intake of high-calorie, high-fat meats.

- **Diabetes**: Vegetarian diets can help manage and prevent type 2 diabetes by improving blood sugar control and increasing insulin sensitivity.

2. **Potential Deficiencies**:

- **Vitamin B12**: Since B12 is primarily found in animal products, vegetarians need to consume fortified foods or supplements to avoid deficiency.

- **Iron**: Plant-based iron is less easily absorbed than iron from meat, so vegetarians need to consume iron-rich foods along with vitamin C to enhance absorption.

- **Omega-3 Fatty Acids**: These are found in high amounts in fish, so vegetarians should consider flaxseeds, chia seeds, and walnuts as alternative sources.

- **Protein**: Although obtainable from plants, vegetarians need to ensure they consume a variety of protein sources to get all essential amino acids.

Environmental Impact

1. **Resource Use**:

   - **Land**: Plant-based diets require less agricultural land compared to diets rich in animal products, reducing deforestation and habitat destruction.

- **Water**: Producing plant-based foods generally uses less water than producing meat, especially beef.

- **Energy**: Growing plants for direct human consumption typically requires less energy than raising livestock.

2. **Greenhouse Gas Emissions**:

- **Lower Emissions**: Vegetarian diets produce fewer greenhouse gases (GHGs) compared to diets high in meat. Livestock farming is a significant contributor to methane and nitrous oxide emissions, both potent GHGs.

- **Climate Change Mitigation**: By reducing reliance on animal agriculture, vegetarian diets can help mitigate climate change and its associated impacts.

3. **Biodiversity**:

- **Preservation**: Reducing meat consumption can alleviate pressure on wild populations and ecosystems, leading to better preservation of biodiversity.

1. **Digestive Health**:

   - **Fiber Intake**: High fiber content in vegetarian diets promotes healthy digestion, regular bowel movements, and a reduced risk of colorectal cancer.

   - **Gut Microbiota**: A plant-based diet can lead to a more diverse and healthy gut microbiota, which is linked to improved overall health.

2. **Energy Levels and Mood**:

   - **Steady Energy**: A balanced vegetarian diet can provide steady energy levels throughout the day due to complex carbohydrates and consistent blood sugar levels.

- **Mental Health**: Some studies suggest that plant-based diets can be associated with better mood and lower levels of depression and anxiety, possibly due to higher intake of antioxidants, vitamins, and minerals.

3. **Longevity**:

- **Life Expectancy**: Some research indicates that vegetarians may have a longer life expectancy due to lower rates of chronic diseases and healthier lifestyles overall.

Adopting a vegetarian diet can offer numerous health benefits, reduce environmental impact, and positively affect bodily functions. However, it requires careful planning to ensure all nutritional needs are met. The shift to plant-based eating can contribute significantly to sustainability efforts and personal well-being.

Navigating social situations as a vegetarian can sometimes be challenging, especially in environments where meat-eating is the norm. Here are some suggestions to help you overcome these challenges with confidence and ease:

1. Communicate Your Dietary Choices

- **Be Clear and Honest**: When dining out or attending social events, let the host or organizer know about your dietary preferences in advance. This allows them to accommodate your needs or give you a heads-up about the menu.

- **Explain Your Reasons**: If someone questions your choice, be prepared to explain your reasons calmly and clearly. Whether it's for health, ethical, environmental, or personal reasons, sharing your perspective can foster understanding.

2. Be Prepared

- **Bring a Dish**: If you're going to a potluck or dinner party, offer to bring a vegetarian dish. This ensures you have something to eat and also introduces others to delicious vegetarian options.

- **Snack Wisely**: Carry some vegetarian snacks with you, like nuts, fruits, or energy bars, in case suitable options are limited.

3. Navigate Dining Out

- **Research Menus**: Before heading to a restaurant, check the menu online to see if they have vegetarian options. If not, call ahead to ask if they can accommodate your needs.

- **Be Flexible**: Sometimes, you might need to get creative with the menu. Don't hesitate to ask if the chef can modify a dish to make it vegetarian.

4. Handle Social Pressure

- **Stay Firm**: If someone tries to pressure you into eating meat, stay firm in your decision. A simple, "No, thank you," is often enough.

- **Use Humor**: Light-hearted humor can diffuse tension. A witty comment like, "I'm on a strict plant-based diet – my vegetables are depending on me!" can keep the mood light.

5. Educate and Advocate

- **Share Information**: If people are genuinely curious about vegetarianism, share information and resources. Recommend books, documentaries, or websites that explain the benefits of a vegetarian diet.

- **Lead by Example**: Sometimes the best way to advocate for vegetarianism is by showing how easy and enjoyable it can be. Invite friends to a vegetarian meal or share your favorite recipes.

6. Build a Support Network

- **Find Like-Minded Friends**: Surround yourself with people who understand and respect your choices. Join vegetarian or vegan groups, both online and offline, to find support and share experiences.

- **Support Non-Vegetarian Friends**: Show respect for others' dietary choices as well. Building mutual respect can lead to more understanding and less conflict.

7. Deal with Misunderstandings

- **Stay Calm and Polite**: If someone makes a mistake or offers you non-vegetarian food, respond politely. A simple, "Thanks, but I don't eat meat," usually suffices.

- **Correct Gently**: If someone spreads misinformation about vegetarianism, gently correct them with facts. Educating others can help reduce misconceptions.

8. Celebrate Your Choice

- **Focus on the Positive**: Celebrate the benefits of your vegetarian lifestyle. Whether it's improved health, environmental impact, or animal welfare, keeping the positives in mind can help you stay committed.

- **Share Your Joy**: Share your passion for vegetarianism by hosting vegetarian dinner parties or sharing your culinary creations on social media.

By following these suggestions, you can confidently navigate social challenges and enjoy your vegetarian lifestyle. Remember, your dietary choices are a personal journey, and it's important to stay true to your values while fostering understanding and respect in your social circles.

Conclusion: Embracing the Vegetarian Journey

Transitioning to a vegetarian diet is more than just a change in what we eat; it's a profound shift in our relationship with food, our bodies, and the world around us. As we conclude this journey, it's essential to reflect on the transformative power of our choices and the myriad benefits they bring.

Choosing a vegetarian lifestyle is a testament to our commitment to health, compassion, and sustainability. Through the pages of this book, we've explored the nutritional advantages of a plant-based diet, delved into the ethical considerations of our food choices, and examined the positive environmental impact of reducing meat consumption. Each step along the way has illuminated the interconnectedness of our actions and their far-reaching effects.

The journey to vegetarianism is unique for each individual. It may begin with a single meal or a conscious decision to explore new culinary horizons. It involves learning, experimenting, and sometimes facing challenges. Yet, every choice we make in favor of plant-based eating is a step towards a healthier and more compassionate world.

By embracing a vegetarian diet, we are not only nourishing our bodies but also nurturing our souls. The vibrant colors, diverse textures, and rich flavors of plant-based foods invite us to celebrate the abundance of nature. They remind us that food is not just sustenance but a source of joy, connection, and creativity.

As we move forward, let us carry with us the wisdom and insights gained from this journey. Let us continue to make mindful choices, seek out new recipes, and share the joy of vegetarian living with others. Let us be ambassadors of a lifestyle that honors the earth and all its inhabitants.

Remember, the transition to a vegetarian diet is not a destination but an ongoing journey. It evolves with us, growing richer and more rewarding with each passing day. By staying open to new experiences, educating ourselves, and fostering a supportive community, we can sustain this journey for a lifetime.

In closing, let us celebrate our progress and look forward to the possibilities that lie ahead. The decision to adopt a vegetarian lifestyle is a powerful one, capable of creating ripples of positive change. Together, we can cultivate a future where health, compassion, and sustainability are at the heart of our dietary choices.

Thank you for embarking on this journey. May your path be

filled with delicious discoveries, vibrant health, and the deep

satisfaction that comes from living in harmony with your

values

A Note of Gratitude to Our Readers

Dear Readers,

As we reach the conclusion of this journey together, I want to take a moment to express my deepest gratitude to each of you. Your decision to pick up this book and explore the path of a vegetarian lifestyle is a testament to your openness, curiosity, and commitment to making mindful choices.

Writing this book has been an incredibly rewarding experience, and knowing that it has found its way into your hands fills me with immense joy. Whether you are at the beginning of your vegetarian journey or have been living this lifestyle for years, your dedication to learning, growing, and embracing a more compassionate way of eating is truly inspiring.

I hope the insights, tips, and recipes shared within these pages have provided you with valuable guidance and inspiration. Transitioning to a vegetarian diet is a significant step, and I am honored to have been a part of your journey. Your willingness to consider new ideas, try new foods, and make conscious choices contributes to a healthier, more sustainable world for all of us.

Thank you for allowing me to be a part of your story. Your support and engagement mean the world to me. I encourage you to continue exploring, experimenting, and sharing your experiences with others. Together, we can create a community that celebrates health, compassion, and sustainability.